Breastfeeding

*A New Mom's Comprehensive
Guide to Breastfeeding*

THIRD EDITION

By: Misty Jordyn

Misty Jordyn

Table of Contents

Misty Jordyn

Introduction

I want to thank you and congratulate you for purchasing the book, "The Breastfeeding Guide". But more than anything, I want to congratulate you for deciding to breastfeed your child. There is so much fulfillment and joy with breastfeeding. Likewise, there will also be a lot of trials, but you will be so proud of yourself once you have succeeded. This book contains proven steps and strategies on how to successfully breastfeed your child minutes after being born up until the weaning years.

Breastfeeding is a very natural thing for mothers to do but unfortunately, it is not instinctive. Many mothers, especially first time moms, struggle to perfect the baby's latch on the breast, feel pain while the baby is feeding, get sores and blisters, think they don't have milk, and other struggles related to feeding. The truth is they simply lack the information and support every breastfeeding mother should have.

First time mothers especially need this book in order to breastfeed their child successfully. Many mothers today get the false impression that breastfeeding is not important because there are other alternatives to feeding such as giving formula milk. What they are not aware of is that babies will only get the most perfect and complete nutrition from their mother's milk and nothing else, at least for the first 6 months of life. The reason why many babies today are prone to sickness is because they have been given artificial food from infancy as opposed to natural mother's milk. If you are serious about giving your child the best nutrition in the world, then be firm about breastfeeding at least for the first 6 months of life and continue on with nutritious supplementary feeding.

With this book, mothers will learn the proper prenatal diet and nutrition, learn how to feed a few minutes or hours after the baby arrives, how often should a baby be fed, what not to feed them during lactation period, how to properly express breast milk, proper breast milk storage and even relactation tips. Get ready mommies because you need to learn, learn, and learn! And we hope you get a hold of this book before the little bundle of joy arrives so you will be well informed. Breastfeeding is very challenging but the rewards will be outstanding.

Thanks again for choosing this book, I hope you enjoy it!

Chapter 1

Natural Foods for Better Milk Production

Breastfeeding is a very beautiful, wonderful, and natural thing. But what most mothers do not know is that breastfeeding will take a lot of work. It can drain your energy and make you feel always hungry. Helping your body to constantly produce a lot of milk during the entire lactation period will also be a challenge. Thus, it is important to prepare your body for breastfeeding. This starts with eating the right food even before you give birth and especially during lactation period. There will be a lot of supplements available in the market that promise to help increase milk supply but why go for the artificial when eating natural food will be better for both you and your child.

That being said here are a few of the most recommended natural foods to eat to help increase milk production and for your body to produce the best quality milk for the baby.

Water

Yes, you read it correct. Not one your fancy health drinks or nutritional supplement, but plain simple water is highly important for milk production. Keep hydrated by aiming to drink at least 8 glasses of water a day, but more is actually required for lactating mothers. Recent studies have shown that the 8 glasses do not need to be water alone but a combination of liquids from natural juices, water contained in fruits and other beverages. However, water is the most beneficial. You can monitor your body's water needs by checking the color of your urine. The color should be light yellow. Darker yellow means you need to drink more water. Breastfeeding mothers should always drink water or natural juices during or after every breastfeeding session. The component of breast milk is 80 percent water so it is but natural for the mother to feel extremely thirsty after feeding sessions as liquids are passed on to the infant.

Plain oatmeal

There are a lot of flavored oatmeal choices in the market but what is recommended is plain oatmeal such as steel cut oats, old-fashioned oats and whole grain oats. You don't need to be told how good oatmeal is for your body. Oatmeal is nutritious, helps lower cholesterol, maintains a healthy blood pressure, helps regulate blood sugar levels and most importantly, helps lactating mothers relax, which increases their oxytocin levels and increase milk supply. Have a bowl every morning and you can also have it in the evenings as it can help you better.

Moringa oleifera

Also commonly known as drumstick tree, horseradish tree, or simply Moringa, has long been widely used in Asia as a very effective lactogenic plant. The leaves can be added soups, vegetable dishes or used for making tea. Moringa leaves contain minerals, vitamins and glycosides. You can make a curry out of it and the leaves can be boiled in water and the water can be cooled and consumed. It can be a bitter and you can add in a little honey and consume it.

Salmon fish

Again, we all know how important it is to consume fish for an overall balanced diet. Salmon meat is packed full of Omega3 and essential fatty acids that is highly nutritious for lactating mothers, thus helping the body produce more milk. Additionally, essential fatty acids are one of the major components of breast milk, which can be obtained in salmon meat. However, it will be essential to check if the fish has any mercury traces, which can be bad for both yours and your baby's health.

Brown rice

This whole grain is full of complex carbohydrates beneficial for breastfeeding mothers to help supplement their growing energy needs. Research has shown that brown rice helps increase production of serotonin in the brain, a neurotransmitter that help in the regulation of mood, appetite and secretion of prolactin which is a hormone responsible for lactation. You can make a simple pilaf out of it or it can also be cooked and added to salads. If you are finding it tough to find brown rice, then you can look for it online.

Asparagus

Rich in Vitamins A, K, C and folic acid, asparagus is also packed full of phytoestrogens that helps in the production of mother's milk. Just like brown rice, it also contains tryptophan, which aids in the secretion of the prolactin hormone, which is also a factor for better milk production. Asparagus can be cooked and added to curries. You can also partially cook it and add it to salads.

Alfalfa

Alfalfa is a plant, which possesses several health benefits. The plant's leaves are used and it is said to contain lots of estrogen. This helps in the production of breast milk. Alfalfa is also rich in multiple vitamins, minerals and other nutrients, which can help supplement a woman's needs after childbirth. Alfalfa sprouts are available at markets and can be added to salads and soups. Seeds are also available, which can be toasted and added to the same. The plant is also available in capsule form, and can be consumed daily with a glass of warm milk.

Fenugreek

Rich in nutrients such as iron, vitamins and minerals, fenugreek seeds are said to be extremely effective in increasing breast milk. It has been used several centuries to help increase the quantity and quality of breast milk and as per doctors, adding a few seeds to everyday foods can help in increasing breast milk within a week's time.

The seeds can be toasted and added to salads or soups and the leaves can be turned into curries. You can also make a tea out of the leaves and consume it with a little sugar added in.

Cumin

Cumin seeds are great for digestion and contain lots of nutrients. The seeds are used most and are quite popular in Asian cuisine. Consuming a few seeds is known to increase the level of breast milk and also helps in curing gastric problems, loose motions and nausea. It is also used to help women gain energy after giving birth. Cumin can be added to curries and the seeds can be boiled in water and the water can be cooled and consumed. A digestive drink can be made by using boiled cumin water, asafetida, mint, salt and pepper.

Nuts

Nuts are rich in multiple nutrients and each one can be consumed for its unique taste. Cashews and almonds are said to be the most preferred nuts to be consumed and can be chopped and added to salads. Walnuts are also equally preferred and so are groundnuts. Powdered almonds can be added to hot milk and consumed on a daily basis. Other nuts can also be powdered and added to milk along with a little turmeric powder.

Breastfeeding women can also consume an energy bar made from nuts, as a snack.

Holy basil

The holy basil is a plant that is better known as Tulsi and is native to India. The herb is said to be extremely effective in providing relief from common colds and coughs and is also known to increase the production of breast milk. It also helps in the smooth movement of the milk and the baby will be able to draw it better. One of the best ways to consume these leaves is by adding it to soups or by chopping it finely and adding it to salads. You can also add a few leaves to a pot of boiling water and allow it to release its entire flavor. Strain the liquid, cool and consume.

Sesame

Sesame seeds are rich in calcium and are used to increase milk supply. Sesame seeds can be toasted and added to salads and they can also be used in curries and to sprinkle over any dish, especially sweets. They can also be used to make breads and just a handful can be consumed every morning and ingested with a glass of water. One great way of using them is to take equal measures sesame seeds and palm sugar and placing the latter in pan and adding the former in after it completely melts. After cooling it, the mix can be shaped into balls and consumed.

Fennel

Fennel seeds and vegetable contain loads of phytoestrogens. These are known to increase the production of breast milk; however, they might also cause a decrease in production, if consumed in excess.

Another use of the seeds and plant is that, they help in reducing the production of gas and aids in digestion. You can toast it a little and add to salads and the vegetable can be used to add to burgers or salads. The vegetable is also great to make a soup out of and the seeds can be boiled in hot water and the water can be cooled and consumed.

Dandelion

Dandelion is a plant, which produces fibrous flowers. It is considered to be a weed but possess several health benefits. It can be used to regain energy after giving birth. It can be used to improve milk production and flow. The flowers are most preferred but all parts of the plant are edible. You can boil the flowers, cool it and consume, or add the leaves to salads and soups. The roots are also quite effective and can be sautéed and added to salads or used in curries and dishes.

Red vegetables

All colored vegetables have a certain quality, which makes them unique and nutritious. All red colored and skinned vegetables are rich in iron and beta-carotene, which helps in improving the formation of breast milk. Some of the best red colored vegetables include carrots, beetroot, sweet potato and red leafed vegetables. Carrot seeds are one of the best options for you to try, as they can help improve the flow of milk. You can add it to your salad by roughly toasting them for a couple of minutes. You make a soup out of beetroot, carrot and sweet potato and consume it on a daily basis.

Flax seed oil

Flax seeds are said to be quite potent in increasing the level of progesterone in women. The seeds are packed with energy and are not as heavy as butter, vegetable oil or any other fat. Flax seeds can be toasted and consumed after being powdered, as the whole seed is not digestible. It is also important to toast the seeds as they can contain chemicals. You can add flax seed oil to salads, soups etc. It can also be used to add to curries, as it is light and can be used in place of regular oils.

Note: These are all safe to be consumed but you might have to check with your doctor first as they might cause an irritation and affect both you and your baby. You might also have to ask if you can have these along with any medication that you are on.

Chapter 2

Foods to avoid

Many times, in spite of being extremely careful, new mothers might end up consuming foods that might affect their breast milk. The doctor might have forgotten to mention certain foods that should not be consumed, and by consuming them, you might be causing your infant problems. The production of milk might not be the only thing being affected and your baby might be having stomach problems owing to what you are consuming.

In this segment, I highlight the tops foods that should be avoided, when you are breastfeeding your child.

Coffee/ tea

Coffee and tea is loaded with caffeine and it is potent enough in travelling through your breast milk to your baby. The caffeine might cause babies to have sleepless nights. It might also cause them to have excessive energy, as they may not be able to burn away the caffeine as much as adults can.

Sodas

Sodas are bad, as they will contain lots of carbon di oxide and chemicals. All of it can seep through breast milk and cause your baby a stomach upset. It is best you drink plain or fruit infused water with your meals. You can also consume plain fruit juices or nutty milks, as they will help improve the quality and quantity of milk you produce.

Alcohol

It should not come as a surprise that you are not supposed to drink alcohol while breastfeeding. Sometimes, after not having a drink for 9 months, mothers might start binging on it. This will affect your breast milk production and also cause your baby discomfort. It might cause him/ her to go into deep sleep and always remain sleepy. If you must, then you can have just one glass of wine every now and then and nothing more.

Chocolate

Chocolates are just as potent as coffees and teas to cause fussiness in babies. If you think that chocolate will only help your baby be happy, then that is a big misconception. If your baby is having problems, then you can try cutting out all forms of chocolate from your diet including drinking chocolate and other such forms of chocolate.

Citrus fruits

Citric fruits such as oranges, grapes and lemons can cause babies to have bad stomachs. These chemicals can be quite potent and seep through the breast. They can cause babies to throw up and cause them to turn irritable. There are also cases of mother's complaining of their babies having developed diaper rashes. Some other fruits, which need to be avoided as much as possible, include mangoes, papayas and pineapple.

Broccoli

Many doctors don't advice lactating mothers to consume broccoli or cauliflower. This is because both contain chemicals, which can seep through the mother's milk and affect the baby's digestion. It might cause the baby to have gas problems and sleepless nights. It is best you avoid consuming any form of the vegetable to avoid problems.

Spices

Spices and spicy foods are a big no-no and I am sure you know about it. But it is important to understand that even very small amounts are enough to cause your baby an upset stomach. You must ideally avoid all types of chilies and if you wish to have something spicy, then add in lemon juice or ginger. These will allow you to get the right amount of heat and not affect your breast milk.

Garlic

Garlic has a very pungent taste and one that is quite strong. The taste might prove to be very strong for a baby, as the flavors will most definitely seep in through the milk. Your baby might not even be interested in sucking and try to avoid drinking if he/ she detect the smell of garlic. If you must, then you can consume garlic infused oil, which might not be strong enough to affect milk.

Raw egg

Raw eggs are a big no-no when it comes to breast-feeding women. Raw eggs can contain e coli and salmonella, both of which might filter through breast milk and enter the body of the baby, which you don't want to experience. It is best to completely avoid eggs, as there might be an egg allergy running in the family. If you do wish to eat then you can boil the egg and allow the yellow to turn powdery. You can also make an omelet out of it or consume scrambled eggs.

Fish

When you breastfeed, you must consider every small detail that is a part of your diet, as you will be completely and directly responsible for what you give your child. You should be careful in choosing the fish, as there might be traces of mercury in it. These days, most water bodies are polluted and you must check with your supermarket and find out where the fish came from. The best seafood to consume is shrimp, as it is quite low in mercury. Shrimps must also be cooked as raw shrimp might cause an allergic reaction.

Chapter 3

Natural Ways to Increase Breast Milk Production

It is very important for a lactating mother to always feel relaxed mentally and physically in order to breastfeed successfully. It might not seem like a woman's body can get affected by certain factors but there can be several things that can affect it.

This is why it is very important to get extra help around the house and to get the full support of the people around her. It is said that women can be super humans and capable of taking on more than they can handle. But sometimes, even super humans require help and it will be useful to have people around to help her out.

> ➢ Mothers need to be physically strong to be able to feed the baby and carry him/ her around. Giving birth can be a very taxing activity and one that will require the woman to be as strong as possible. The only way she can attain it is through the consumption of good food and lots of clean water to drink.

> ➢ Apart from physical fitness, she also needs to be mentally happy. Stress can significantly affect the ability of the mother to produce milk.

- Breastfeeding is connected to the mother's brain because it signals the body to produce milk for the baby.

- If she is under immense stress, then in spite of wanting to produce milk, she might not be able to. She might have worries and tensions, which might be causing her subconscious to take over.

- One way for the mother to remain calm and composed is to indulge in a little meditation. It will allow her to take mind off of the ongoing chaos and allow her to relax and recoil. It will also help her in being happy and as per some experts, a happy mother can pass the happiness to her baby through the milk that she produces and feeds.

- Lactation experts often advise that drinking warm tea, warm soup or even just sipping warm water will help increase breast milk production. Warm soups and drinks help the body relax and also increases liquid intake.

- This tea needs to be herbaceous tea such as dandelion or minty and not regular caffeine laden teas. It is best that thee tea be prepared fresh every time and not be placed in flasks.

- The freshest of vegetables and other ingredients should be used, as it will be important for the mother to get the best, nutritious food.

- Along with these, it is best that the mother get adequate sleep. Sleeping long hours allows the body to repair both physically and mentally. This rest and sleep should be extra and different from an 8-hour nightly sleep.

➢ Another way to increase breast milk is to have the infant latch directly to the breast. The baby's sucking stimulates the nerves in the breast making it produce more milk.

➢ Feeding often also helps increase milk supply. It is recommended to feed a small infant every 2 hours so the baby's blood sugar levels won't drop.

➢

The science behind milk production

Many women wonder how their breasts produce milk. This can be a very good question and pursuing its answer will help new mothers feed their babies better.

Women's breasts are known as mammary glands and they are exclusively meant to produce milk for infants. This milk is vital for both the mother and the baby and contains lots of vitamins and nutrients that help the baby grow strong and healthy.

Each breast consists of a lot of components and they are explained as under

- Mammary gland: The mammary gland or breast gland is responsible for the up keep of breast health and releases hormones that aid in producing the milk.

- Connective tissue: The connective tissue is a set of tissues that help in binding the breast tissues together and are responsible for giving the breast's their shape.

- Adipose tissue: The adipose tissue is meant to protect the breasts from injury and they are responsible for determining a woman's breast size. They, however, will not determine the quantity or quality of milk that the woman produces.

- Lymph tissue: The lymph tissue is a clear tissue that supplies the breast with a cleansing liquid. It helps in flushing out any impurities and toxins from the breast. The lymph also helps in supplying the breast with healthy cells that combat diseases and keep the breast healthy.

- Nerves: The nerves that are present in the breasts are extremely sensitive and they are responsible for the breast to produce milk. When the baby latches and suckles, the nerves signal the breasts to produce and supply more milk.

- Blood: The blood present inside the breasts contains plasma, red blood cells and white blood cells and is responsible for supplying fresh oxygen, nutrients and disease combating cells to breasts. The blood also assists in removing out the toxins and impurities. A rush of blood to the breast causes them to produce more milk and this generally happens when the baby is nursing.

- Alveoli cells: These cells are situated inside the lobe of the breast and secrete the milk. This milk then travels to the nipple pores through the milk ducts. The nipple has multiple pores through which the milk is secreted.

What your partner can do

A baby is not just the mother's responsibility and although she will be more than happy to tend to her baby's needs, it is also important for the father to contribute, equally, towards taking care of the baby.

The father can only do a little, physically, when it comes to nursing the baby, but he can provide emotional support to the mother. He can also help in holding the baby while nursing and if there are twins or multiples, then the father has to dedicate a lot of time and effort in helping the mother nurse the children.

Your partner must take care of your baby, or babies, when you need to rest as lots of rest and relaxation is vital for good milk production. There is some scientific evidence to prove that the husband sitting next to his wife while she feeds their baby helps in spreading love and warmth and allows them to gel as a family.

Fitness for breast feeding mothers

Many women think that exercising will affect their quality of milk and decide to stay low. But this is a misconception. The mother's fitness is of extreme relevance when it comes to her producing good quality and quantity milk.

Although you might not be able to start exercising immediately after giving birth or even a month later, you can start taking walks and slowly move towards performing light exercises in a couple of months.

You can ask your doctor the exact time when you can start to exercise and decide on a routine that you can follow.

Some women prefer aerobics, as it will help your body attain a good amount of exercise and not tire you out. The same applies to swimming, and it can be quite therapeutic as well.

Make sure you buy appropriate clothing for your exercise sessions and might have to wear a padded bra to help conceal any milk leak. You can pump out as much as you can or nurse your baby and then exercise, to help preserve as much milk as possible.

You can get your partner to join you during exercise or find a group of women who are also on a post pregnancy- fitness spree.

Chapter 4

Breastfeeding Your Child

It is often a misconception that milk will automatically come when the baby arrives. But this only happens to a few gifted women who are overflowing with milk even before they give birth. Most often, the scenario is that the mother will panic because she does not see milk coming out of her breast. The truth is, for the first few days after a mother gives birth, milk does not always arrive. What does come out is what you call 'colostrum', often called the first milk, and is exactly what a newborn baby needs, not the milk. Most mothers don't even know she is producing it because it only comes out in small amounts. It is often produced a few months during pregnancy and sometimes leaks out having a yellowish color. This is the first milk that infants are supposed to get and it is not supposed to be a lot. A baby's stomach upon birth is only about the size of a small grape and only needs very little amount of nourishment.

The first milk

Colostrum is often referred to as 'beestings', or simply 'first milk'. Colostrum is full of immunoglobulin and antibodies that an infant needs to cope with the outside world. It will help protect the baby from viruses, bacteria, and will help them expel the meconium or the first stools, which is blackish in color. Think of this as your baby's first line of defense - their first vaccine. Babies who were able to acquire colostrums from their mother usually have a stronger immune system. Colostrum that comes out of the mother's breast for the first 3 days to 1 week is very important for the baby. This will be yellowish in color. After a week or two, the white milk will finally start to come out, so the mother should expect to feed the baby more.

The proper latch

The way the baby's mouth latches on to the breast is very important. First of all, it ensures that the baby will be getting sufficient milk. Proper latch better stimulates the breast so it will produce more milk. When a baby is latched on properly, the mother should not feel any pain while breastfeeding. Any discomfort is usually remedied by correcting the baby's latch. How can you tell if the baby is latched on properly? The baby's nose should be free to breathe and the head should be tipped back a little. A bigger area of the areola should be visible on the upper lip of the infant than the lower lip. To achieve a perfect latch, make sure the baby's mouth is wide open before attaching to the breast. The tongue should be positioned at the bottom of the breast with the chin touching the breast. Hold the baby in a comfortable position and use pillows when necessary.

Pumping breast milk

Direct latching is not the only option when it comes to breastfeeding an infant. Even working mothers who need to leave their children for several hours can still give their child breast milk by pumping. This can be done by hand express or with the use of a breast pump. There are different kinds of breast pumps available in the market ranging from a manual pump to the more pricey electric pumps. Pumping on a regular schedule can also help increase breast milk production. However, pumping is not recommended for the first 6 weeks after giving birth. This is the time when milk supply has not yet been established. Pumping will only tell the brain to produce more milk at a very early stage, which can lead to over supply or over production of milk. This can have adverse effects such as frequent engorgements that can lead to mastitis (more about this on the next chapter).

Foremilk and hind milk

A mother's breast milk is perfect because it can provide everything that the baby needs. This is evident with the production of foremilk and hind milk. Mothers who pump their milk will notice that the first milk that will come out of their breast is almost watery. This is called the foremilk. After a few minutes of pumping, the milk will gradually become white and thicker and that is called the hind milk. The foremilk has water content to satisfy the infant's thirst while the hind milk is filled with fat content that provides nourishment and energy for the young one.

Chapter 5

Problems You Might Encounter

As you already know by now, breastfeeding is not easy. Some mothers may be lucky enough not to experience any problems once they have mastered the proper latch but to the vast majority, there will be different hurdles. Problems encountered during breastfeeding is one of the main reasons why some mothers give up and resort to alternative measures such as giving formula milk. The fact is that they simply lack the information and knowledge on how to handle these hurdles.

Here are some of the most common problems breastfeeding mother's encounter and possible solutions:

Sore nipples

This could be due to a number of things but the most common reason is a shallow latch. The nipples may feel tender, sensitive and the baby's latching may be painful. Others can even have blisters making feeding even more painful and difficult. When this happens, check if the baby's latch is correct. You may also try to pump the blistered breast while allowing the baby to latch on the good breast. You are advised to not apply anything that you think is suspicious to cure the problem. One form of instant relief is to rub a little ice over it and it will help in flattening the blisters. You can apply a little milk cream over the blisters, as it will not affect the baby or your milk and help provide relief from the problem.

Engorgement

Engorged breasts happen when it has not been emptied for the recommended time and it starts to feel extremely full, firm, swollen and painful. It can be accompanied by a slight fever and the pain can extend up to the armpits. This usually happens a week after giving birth as more blood flows into the breast tissues getting it ready to produce more milk after the colostrum production. It may last for several days but will eventually go away. To ease the pain, let your baby latch on and feed longer to empty the breast. Apply hot compress to lessen the pain and encourage milk flow. Massage the breasts and pump or hand express to let the milk out. You can also massage the breasts while your baby is feeding to ensure that the milk will come out and flow more efficiently.

Mastitis

This is an inflammation on the tissues of the breast that has become an infection. The breast will feel sore and swollen and may also be accompanied with flu like symptoms such as fever, headaches and muscle soreness. You may also develop a clogged milk duct, which will feel like a lump on the breast. To relieve the symptoms, certain painkillers can be taken such as paracetamol. Get some rest, don't wear tight-fitting clothes, breastfeed more frequently and apply warm compress on the breasts. If the symptoms do not improve, see a doctor. Do not start taking any other medicines such as antibiotics because it might not be recommended for breastfeeding mothers.

Biting

Some infants, especially the ones that are teething, can start to bite at your nipple and it can cause you immense pain. To help them understand that it is wrong to do so, you can put your little finger in their mouth and free them from your breast and say "NO". Make sure you don't shout but be as firm and affirmative as possible. If your baby still bites, then you can immediately stop feeding and lay him or her down. This will make them realize that biting you will evoke a negative response and they will stop immediately. If your baby is big enough, then you can give them teething toys or use a pacifier to help ease their teething aches.

Blocked milk ducts

Breastfeeding mothers may feel a lump in the breast accompanied with soreness, pain, and a reddish tender patch on the skin. Clogged milk ducts may be an early sign of mastitis. This happens if the baby is not fully draining the milk from the breast or when you are producing milk much faster than the baby is consuming it. The milk that is left behind the duct is being forced out into the tissues causing inflammation and swelling. To relieve symptoms of clogged milk ducts, apply warm compress and gently massage the area around the lump. You can fill a muslin cloth with some sea salt, heat it on a griddle and gently place it over it. Feed longer to help fully drain the milk.

Low milk supply

It is a common misconception that a mother is not able to produce milk. Unless there are medical reasons involved, almost all mothers are capable of producing an abundant supply of milk. It is normal for a mother not to see milk flowing out of her breast on the first few days after giving birth. This is because colostrum is produced by the body instead of milk, which is exactly what the baby needs. The milk flow will start to be visible a week after giving birth. This is when you might experience engorgement and leaking breasts. But even when your milk doesn't leak out or doesn't come out when you press upon your breast, rest assured that your baby is getting it during a direct latch. The evidence that your baby is getting enough milk is by the wet diapers and yellowish poop. To help increase milk production, eat lactogenic foods (as discussed in the first chapter of this book). Feed on demand or pump on a regular schedule because this will signal the body to produce more milk for the baby. Drink liquids before and after every feed and hydrate yourself throughout the day.

When you encounter other problems related to your breastfeeding or your child's feeding habits, do not give up breastfeeding. Instead, seek the advice of a lactation expert, a midwife, a pediatrician or your OB gynecologist. Your problem might turn out to be very common among breastfeeding moms and the remedy can be very simple. Remember that once your milk supply has been established after about 6 weeks, then breastfeeding will be as easy as pie and you would be an expert by then. You will soon reap the wonderful benefits of breastfeeding for both you and the baby and help him/ her have a healthy life.

Chapter 6

Your Child's Feeding Guide

Mothers should trust their bodies and their capability to produce milk for the baby. The body will produce the perfect milk for their babies. Almost every month, the components of breast milk changes according to the baby's needs. The amount of milk the baby needs changes as well.

The first 6 months

The first 6 months of the baby's life is very crucial for nourishment. The World Health Organization suggest to exclusively breastfeed baby to provide optimum nourishment and protection. Exclusively breastfeeding literally means giving the baby only breast milk for the first 6 months, with no water, vitamins, and solid foods. This is because the baby's digestive function is not yet fully developed to properly break down other sources of nourishment, thus putting strain in their fragile bodies. Breast milk is easily digestible and is perfect for the baby's gut. If worried about the baby's hydration, keep in mind that breast milk is composed of 80 percent water and 20 percent powerful and nutritious food for the baby. This includes immunoglobulin that fight off viruses and bacteria, Lactoferrin, which is an iron-building protein, and Lysozyme, which is an enzyme essential to proper digestive function. Breast milk also contains a much higher percentage of Carnitine, DHA and RHA compared to formula milk. Exclusively breastfeeding the baby for the first 6 months of life helps protect the baby from illnesses, diarrhea, respiratory infections and possible allergies.

The first week: size and volume of your baby's tummy

- ➢ Day 1 5-7 ml (1/2 tsp)Stomach is just the size of a cherry fruit

- ➢ Day 3 22-27 ml (.75 to 1.0 oz) Stomach is just the size of a walnut

- ➢ 1 week 45-60 ml (1.5 to 2 oz) Stomach is just the size of an apricot

- ➢ 1 month 80-150 ml (2.5-5 oz) Stomach is the size of a large egg

How often should a baby feed?

Ideally, a baby should be breastfed on demand. This means allowing the baby to feed as much as he or she wants, day and night. Signs that a baby is hungry include restlessness, sucking on fingers and fists, and opening mouth with head turning from side to side as if looking and trying to reach for the breast.

Aim to breastfeed a newborn baby every 2 to 3 hours. This means feeding for 8 to 12 times a day. If the infant is sleeping at night, gently wake him up and offer some milk. Frequent feeding will help the baby maintain a normal blood glucose level. Breastfeed a baby more frequently when sick to help the baby fight the sickness and recover faster (mother's milk has disease fighting immunity).

Feed for at least 15 to 20 minutes on each breast to ensure that the baby will empty the milk ducts and get to the hind milk, which contains the good fats that the baby needs. As the baby gets older, they become more efficient in feeding and may only take 5 to 10 minutes on each breast.

Starting solids after 6 months

On the 6th month, your baby will be more active and thus needs more good fats and calories to burn. This is the time when complimentary feeding is offered to the child. Continue breastfeeding on demand but offer a variety of other healthy foods, particularly fruits and vegetables. Keep in mind, however, that breast milk should still be the primary source of food at this stage until the baby turns 1 year old. Feeding twice to 3 times a day should be enough at this period.

Chapter 7

Pumping and Storage

Breastfeeding can be very demanding and it would seem like the baby will need the mother 24/7 but there's still a way to exclusively breastfeed a child even if the mother is away. This is by way of expressing milk from the breast and storing it. There are two ways to express milk, one is by hand express and the other is with the use of a breast pump.

Hand expressing breast milk

Prepare a clean storage bottle to catch expressed milk. Wash hands and clean nipples using a warm cloth or cotton ball dipped in warm water. Massage the breasts gently to stimulate tissues and help it produce more milk. Put a gentle pressure on the area around the areola and massage through kneading in order to express the milk. Collect the expressed milk in the storage bottle.

Pumping breast milk

The kind of pump to use will depend on individual preferences. Some may find manual pumps effective while others consider electric pumps more efficient. Manual pumps are relatively cheaper than electric. Many mothers tend to start with trying out several types of manual pumps until they settle to a specific unit. If manual pump don't work for them, they usually move on to buying the more expensive electric pump. Expressing with the use of a breast pump can have its advantage and disadvantages. For those who find it difficult to hand express, pumps can be a more efficient alternative and can express milk faster. But others find it difficult and painful. Excessive use of electric pumps can also damage capillaries in the breast tissues.

After expressing breast milk and you are not yet planning to offer it to the baby, cover the container and place it in a cool area. It is recommended to offer it to the baby within 4 hours (if kept on room temperature of about 25-37 degrees Celsius) or within 8 hours (if kept on room temperature of about 15-25 degrees Celsius). It should not be kept on temperatures above 37 degrees. If planning to build up a stash, so the baby can feed while you are away, storing the milk in a refrigerator or freezer will prolong its life. Here is a milk storage guideline that might be helpful.

Storing breast milk

In an ice box- Keep milk containers tightly closed. Fill with ice placed in a plastic bag so that it won't contaminate the milk bottles when it melts. The milk containers can also be placed in a zip lock bag so that it won't mix with the melted ice. Milk stored in this manner should be good for 24-48 hours.

In the refrigerator- Keep milk containers tightly closed and place in the coldest part of the refrigerator, towards the back. Milk stored in this manner should be good for 3-5 days.

In the ref freezer- Keep milk containers tightly closed, or better yet, use a milk storage bag to save space. When placed in the compartment part of the freezer, milk should be good for 2 weeks. When placed in the freezer part, milk will be good for 3 months.

In the chest freeze- if you have a separate freezer intended for deep-freezing, breast milk will be good to use for 6 months up to a year.

Always label the milk before storing. Place the date and time it was expressed so you will know which batch of milk to use first. Thaw the milk on room temperature before offering to the baby. Never thaw in hot water or place in the microwave, as it will destroy the essential nutrients in the milk. For frozen milk, remove it from the freezer hours before you will use it so that it can thaw on its own. You can place the milk containers on tap or a slightly warm water to help it thaw faster. Once thawed, do not shake the milk. Simply swirl it to break down the white components.

When storing breast milk in colder temperatures, any regular milk bottle can be used. There are also milk storage bottles that can be bought in baby stores and these are reusable. If planning to freeze the milk, it is recommended to use a disposable milk bag to save freezer space and to prevent damage to the milk bottles.

Chapter 8

Breastfeeding When Ill/ After Surgery

Breast feeding your infant can be extremely important for both you and your baby, but it might not always go according to plan. Mothers who are sick and down with an illness, or have had breast surgery after giving birth to their baby, might have to exercise a little precaution while nursing their infant, and these precautionary measures are explained as under

Fever/ cold

For mothers who have a fever or cold, it is safe to continue feeding your baby. Many women don't realize that they would have passed the infection to their infant a couple of days prior to falling sick and chances are the baby is already fighting the germs off.

To help supplement their immune system, you will have to feed them, as your body would have kicked into action to produce anti bodies for your illness. You can pass on these anti bodies, and your child will be able to fight it off better.

You can consume immunity building herbal tablets or capsules to help you ward off the sickness but if the fever lasts for more than 3 days then you can visit both your doctor and your child's pediatrician.

Remember to ask for a medicine or antibiotic that is breastfeeding safe and make sure you follow the course prescribed to you to get better soon.

When you are combating a fever and cold, you must drink as much water as you can and can also consume an isotonic for the salts and sugars in your body to balance out. Consuming fresh vegetables and fruits will allow you to recover faster as also help you produce enough milk for your baby when you are sick.

Stomach ailments/ severe illness

If you are suffering from a bad stomach infection and have loose motions, then you can consider consuming an anti diarrheal like fenugreek seeds. You can churn them and add to water and consume the water every 2 hours and this will help stop the motions as also get rid of the infection.

If this does not work, then you can consult the doctor and ask for something that will not affect your breast milk.

If your baby is also showing discomfort and passing regular motion, then you can ask your pediatrician for help and maybe feed a little of the fenugreek water to help the infection pass out. But this will be extremely rare as breast milk generally cannot pass stomach infections.

If you are down with something more severe and there is no option for you but to consume an anti biotic that is not breast milk friendly, then before starting on the medicines, you can pump enough milk and store it. To help your milk drain, you can pump it all out and discard it, as it will not be fit for your baby to consume.

If you don't get a chance to pump enough before you start the treatment, then you can have your baby consume formula until such time as you are fit to nurse your infant again.

It is advisable that you pump out at least 6 hours of milk after you are off of the antibiotics and ask your doctor if it is safe to, now, administer the milk to your baby.

Dealing with baby's illness

Sometimes, not getting enough breast milk can weaken the baby's immunity and cause them to develop illnesses such as jaundice and reflux, which need to be dealt with to help the baby remain healthy.

- Jaundice is common amongst babies and is mostly brought on because of not having enough breast milk. Their bodies are incapable of flushing out bilirubin and this can cause them to develop the illness.

- It can be harmless for them to develop it after the first month and simply providing them with enough breast milk can help in flushing out the excess bilirubin from the body. The illness will subside within a week's time.

- Many times, the jaundice can be brought on owing to impurities present in the mother's milk and the doctor might advise stopping breast feeding until all the impurities from the mother's body is removed and the bay be put on formula.

- The baby might also have to go through phototherapy for the excess bilirubin is drained from the body and the mother can start feeding again, after the baby is back to being normal.

- Some mothers fear feeding their babies after a jaundice incident but you must remember that you were not responsible for its onset and must not punish yourself and your baby for something that was beyond your control. So don't be too harsh on yourself and do as the doctor instructs you to.

Reflux

- Acid Reflux or better known as gastro esophageal reflux disease (GERD) refers to your baby spitting out or vomiting milk after a few minutes of being fed. This can occur if the muscles that close the stomach open up randomly causing the ingested food to come back to the mouth.

- If this is occurring, then you can wait for a couple of days and see if it subsides. But if the baby continues to spit out milk, then you can consult your doctor.

- The doctor might have to give your baby some medication, which will help him or her regulate their stomach acid and they should improve within a week's time or less.

- Remember that you cannot shift from your milk to formula when your baby is having a reflux as he or she will not be able to digest it well enough. Your breast milk would not have caused the reflux and so, you must continue feeding your baby your milk.

- Some of the other signs and symptoms of GERD that you must be on the lookout for include incessant crying after feeding, writhing and twisting out of pain, not being able to nurse for more than 5 minutes and a refusal to latch to the breast, not having a consistent weight gain, crying at nights and remaining awake at night, effusing to swallow and spitting out milk in a jet stream and the stomach area of the baby feeling hot and burning. You must consult your doctor if any of these persist for more than 2 days.

Breast surgery

- Women with breast surgery can feed their babies, but how often or successfully they can, will depend entirely on the type of surgery that has been done.

- If the woman has had a surgery where the fold under her breast has incisions, then she can feed her baby without any problem. She can choose the other breast if only one has an incision underneath. Once the incision heals, then both breasts can be used to feed the baby.

- If there is an incision across the nipple or areola, then there might be a little pain and discomfort when feeding your baby. But you can solve this problem by applying a little milk cream over the incision to soothe it. You can also choose to pump the milk and feed your baby as pumping might be less painful as compared to feeding your baby directly.

- Women who have breast implants can feed their baby without a problem. Neither the mother nor the baby will be at any risk. If you are not sure, then you can ask your pediatrician for advice.

- But if the surgery has caused for some milk ducts to be removed, then there might be a problem with producing enough milk. You might have to supplement it with formula.

- If you wish to have surgery done due to an emergency, then you can ask your surgeon to maintain as much of the tissue and ducts as possible to help you continue nursing your baby.

Cleft lip or cleft palate

- Many mothers panic at the thought or sight of a cleft lip or palate and wonder if there is something very wrong with their baby's mouth.

- But there is absolutely no need to worry, as a cleft palate or cleft lip is a very common congenital condition and can occur in babies that are premature or did not have enough time for the lip and cleft to develop and form properly.

- This condition is easily treated through surgery and your baby can have a full recovery. But the condition will cause your baby to have problems latching to your breast.

- For this, you can ask the doctor to help you with latching your baby in the correct way and how you can continue feeding them after their surgery.

- Remember that you must feed your baby colostrum, even if he or she has a cleft palate or lip, and if it is impossible for your baby to latch, then you can pump it and feed your baby through a cup.

Chapter 9

Re-lactation Tips

Any woman has the ability to produce milk. This is because the hormones responsible for releasing milk, prolactin and oxytocin, are pituitary hormones. This means that with proper stimulation of the breast and nipples, the brain can send signals to the body to produce milk.

There are different reasons why a woman would want to re lactate. There are mothers who were not able to immediately breastfeed and resorted to formula milk but want to get back to breastfeeding. There are also those who have adopted a child and want to provide the best possible milk for their baby, which is breast milk. However, don't expect it to be an easy process.

Mothers who have delivered a baby within a 3-month period might find more success because their hormone levels are still naturally high. But for mothers who are past this period, the challenge might be greater.

The best possible way to re lactate is to keep breastfeeding via direct latch. The baby's suckling on the nipples is the best stimulant on the nerves in the breast that will signal the brain to produce the milk. Nurse as frequently as possible and accompany that with regular pumping. Invest in a hospital-grade double electric pump. Use it every 2 to 3 hours for at least 15 minutes on each breast. This will help stabilize milk supply. Additionally, keep yourself hydrated, eat lots of lactogenic foods, and keep yourself happy and relaxed at all times. It might be very helpful to seek the advice of a certified lactation consultant to make the process faster and easier.

Don't expect milk to come gushing out. There may only be drops of milk even if you've been feeding and pumping religiously for a few weeks. Re lactation period is different for every woman. Don't give up and focus your mind on producing milk. Remember the three B's when it comes to breastfeeding – brain, breast and baby. How you think will greatly affect milk production. Keep the baby close to you and the breast to encourage the brain to send more signals to the body to produce more milk.

Chapter 10

Benefits of Breastfeeding for Mothers

The benefits of breastfeeding for mothers cannot be underscored enough. In addition to the emotional fulfillment that she derives from the physical and psychological intimacy of nursing, breastfeeding has a calming effect on the mother as much as it has on the baby. These feelings of calm and well-being can be attributed to the release of a complex group of hormones by the body in response to the action of breast-feeding.

A major hormone whose production is triggered by breastfeeding is prolactin. In its simplest description, prolactin is a hormone that triggers milk production in nursing mothers; however various studies all over the world have discovered more than 300 separate effects of prolactin. The benefits of prolactin are truly numerous. As said it stimulates lactation, is responsible for the enlargement of the breasts during this period. Prolactin is also the key hormone in providing sexual gratification; it does this by acting as a sort of counterbalance to the effects of another hormone, dopamine, which in turn is responsible for sexual arousal.

Another major hormone whose role cannot be stressed enough is Oxytocin. This is a hormone whose benefits are as complex in nature as its structure and composition. IN fact this is perhaps the hormone that defines the notions of intimacy in our body. These properties come to fore during and after childbirth. During the period of childbirth, secretion of this hormone results in distention of the cervix, thereby facilitating trouble free childbirth. After the delivery, this very hormone plays the defining role in generating the feeling of maternal intimacy and bonding. And during the breastfeeding phase, stimulation of nipples by the suckling baby results in secretion of this hormone, which in turn triggers lactation. Hence you can see how Oxytocin is one of those most important and significant hormones in the human body.

Moving on, let us now look at the benefits of breastfeeding to mothers in detail. We shall go over the points as mentioned below, one by one.

Reduction in risk of breast cancer

There is conclusive scientific evidence to prove that the risks of breast cancer is reduced by almost 25 percentage in women who breastfeed their babies. And this said reduction of risk is directly proportional to the complete duration of breastfeeding by the woman in her lifetime. The more a woman breastfeeds her babies, the lower will be her chances of getting breast cancer.

Reduction in risk of uterine and ovarian cancer

As in the case of lower risk of breast cancer, breastfeeding reduces the overall risk of uterine and ovarian cancer. Many researchers have opined that this is due to the fact that during the period of breastfeeding, a woman's body produces very less amounts of estrogen. It is believed that with lower levels of Estrogen, there won't be enough of that hormone to line the walls of the uterus. This lining is considered to be the key reasons for cancerous growth in the uterus.

Lesser chances of Osteoporosis

Osteoporosis is a progressive bone disease, the major symptoms of which are reduction of bone density and bone mass. This makes the bones and joints more prone to fracture. It is very common in women who are in their menopausal or postmenopausal stage, and this kind osteoporosis is called Type-1 or postmenopausal osteoporosis. A number of studies are clearly showing that women who breastfeed after childbirth run a markedly lower risk of developing type-1 osteoporosis after menopause. To this end, they also seem to have very low chances of hip fracture and dislocation in their later years.

Helps in child spacing

In today's hectic world and its breathless pace, most couples find it extremely hard to raise more than one child. Some couples plan it in such a way that the first child is old enough to not require the continuous and unbridled attention of a parent when the second child is born. The technique of child spacing comes into picture here. A large number of couples, who desire to have more than one child, prefer the second child to be born at least 3 to 4 years after the first one. The benefits of breastfeeding play a subtle but hugely significant role here.

Breastfeeding delays ovulation naturally and as long as she has a suckling baby, she would remain infertile. Obviously, the woman will not be able to be conceive when she is still breastfeeding. Hence in this case the couples can comfortably plan for a baby after 2 or 3 years, when the woman is ready again. This is a much better and convenient option than artificial means of child spacing which involves birth control and contraception.

Better emotional health

Breastfeeding is as much an emotional thing as it is a physical. As mentioned earlier in this chapter, the release of various "rewarding" hormones, so called because of their action in the brain's reward centers, provides a feeling of bliss to the nursing mother. It puts the mind of the mother at ease and she feels way more settled and content than ever with the suckling baby at her breast. Indeed it can quite very much be the happiest and most content moments in a woman's life and happiness can do wonders to her emotional set up.

Countless studies have proven that the breastfeeding can be a boon for mothers dealing with post partum depression. The emotional satisfaction derived from the process of breastfeeding can be the most effective salve for an anxiety-ridden mind.

Weight loss

Weight gain during pregnancy is a very amusing phenomenon. Amusing because, when the woman is carrying, the weight makes her look glowing and full of health, whereas the same extra pounds can give the image of being fat and blotted after childbirth. Hence it is no wonder that most women are too anxious to shed all that extra inches around the midriff and elsewhere. In some cases this can prove to be a very dangerous tendency as the mother may start on extreme diets with negligible nutritional content.

There are two angles to risk. One is the apparent danger posed to the baby. If the nursing mother is not consuming sufficient, nutrient rich food, it affects the quality of her milk and consequently the health of her baby, whose only source of nutrition is the milk. The second angle is the danger to the mother herself. Insufficient nutrition can take its take its toll on the body and lead to illness.

Breastfeeding is a solution to this conundrum too. Generally breastfeeding mothers are faster than those who don't, in losing the post partum weight within the first month of childbirth. They return back to their pre-pregnancy body weight way quicker than mothers who don't breastfeed.

Cost factor

The cost factor cannot be ignored; especially, considering the burgeoning costs of baby products in the market today.

Breastfeeding doesn't involve 99% of those costs. The formulas that are in the market today are absurdly expensive and overrated and still do not meet the quality of a mother's breast milk. In case of middle-income families, where having a child is as much a financial decision as an emotional and familial one, this is a factor that is impossible to ignore.

Convenience factor

Breastfeeding is immensely convenient and simple as compared to feeding formula foods to the baby. It can be anywhere and anytime. The moment you feel the baby is hungry and needs food, all you need to do is find a private spot and let the baby suckle. Breast milk is warm and perfect for the baby's palate.

Whereas in case of formula foods, you have to mix it in the right proportion, heat it for attaining the right consistency and carry it around in containers wherever you go. And still you stand the chance of feeding cold food to the baby. Cold in temperature and emotion!

Miscellaneous advantages

Now let us look at some miscellaneous convenience factors that breast-feeding has. As mentioned above it is immensely easier to feed your baby from your breast than give it some concoction of grains whipped up in the kitchen. Then there is the freedom it gives you. Go for the get together with your friends, the occasional shopping trip to the mall, the garden party of your neighbors, anywhere you want as long as you feel the environment suits your baby, without a worry about its feeding.

Breast milk is warm and ready for consumption at any time and this really makes it convenient to feed the baby as and when it wants. Night feedings are a lot easier this way because you can feed the baby without getting up from the bed and disrupting the sleep of your partner

Chapter 11

Breastfeeding in Public

Feeding your baby in public places might be a necessity, as you cannot sit at home all day long. You will have to go out and meet people and show off your baby to others. But pulling down your blouse or lifting your top in public can be quite embarrassing, especially if there are men around.

But that should not stop you from doing it, as your child will need to be fed and not feeding him or her might cause them to turn cranky. In order for you to tackle this issue, here are some things that you can do to successfully feed your child in public and not be embarrassed by it.

- The very first thing that you must do is to buy a few comfortable tops that are loose and can be lifted from down with ease. It will allow you to pull your top up easily and slip your baby inside your top and cover his or her head with it. You can also choose a button down shirt as it will be easy for you to unbutton and from top and access your breast. There are special breast feeding tops that can be bought from maternity stores which will have a zipper placed in place of the nipple, which you can easy pull down and allow your baby to suckle.

- Just like the special top, you must buy yourself a bra that has a hook or zipper flap placed over the nipple area, which you can easily undo to access your nipples. But you must buy good quality ones from good brands as poor quality hooks or buttons might cause chaffing of your nipples. You must try it on to check your comfort level and only wear it if you are comfortable in it as you might not be able to change it once you are in public. You can also opt for a boob tube, as it will be easy for you to pull it down while feeding and pull it back up, once you are done.

- If you do not want to wear loose clothes as it might look unflattering, then you can opt for a breast feeding blanket. A breast feeding blanket is a special soft blanket that you can pull over your shoulders and cover your baby's head with it. Make sure you have a nice and soft one as it might rub against your baby's head and make him or her feel uncomfortable. You must have someone to assist you as you might find it tough to wrap it around your shoulders by yourself. If you are not conscious of your look then you can pin the blanket on your shoulders and pull it around you easily.

- You might not always find a place to sit down and feed your baby and to tackle this situation; you can invest in a good baby sling. Baby slings are the most convenient way to carry your baby and you can place your baby inside the sling, facing you. You can then adjust your nipple to help your baby reach it and can feed him or her while walking around. Make sure the sling is affixed properly and try it on before buying one. The material needs to be comfortable and your baby should be securely placed close to your body.

- If there is too much crowd around and you are inside a mall or someplace similar, then you can simply make your way to a change room or a women's lounge and feed your baby. Some women prefer to ask permission and use a changing room to feed their baby as it will be convenient to sit down and feed your baby. But whatever area that you choose, make sure that it is comfortable as you might have to spend 15 to 30 minutes and trying to vacate before fully feeding might make your baby cranky.

- Remember that breast feeding is a legal activity and if there is someone who approaches to object, then you need not stop. There can be people who will approach you and ask you to cover up or try and get you to move to a different location but you need not do any of that and can continue to feed your baby. Several states like New York have legislations laid down which will protect your right to feed your baby. Do it proudly and think of it as educating others around you, especially other young mothers.

- If you are inviting uncomfortable glares, then simply smile back at them. To help you stay put and not vacate, you can carry a copy of the legislation that supports breastfeeding in public and hand it to them. Once they read it, they will not bother you and walk away. You can have a soft copy on your phone or mail and show it to them. If nothing is working and they are forcing you to move, then you can consider calling police for help.

- To help you breast feed smoothly in a public place, you can practice at home. You can sit in front of the mirror and look at how you will appear. You can adjust your position and show as little as your breasts as possible and generally, a nursing baby will be able to cover 90% of your breast. Make sure you are practicing when your baby is nursing and don't force him or her to latch on.

- Lastly, you can always carry a bottle of your pumped milk anywhere that you go. You will be able to feed your baby in case there is no proper place to sit or walk around. Make sure the milk is used within 6 hours of pumping.

These form the various measures that you can adapt to peacefully and efficiently breast feed your child in public.

Chapter 12

Benefits of Breastfeeding in Babies

Nature intended babies to derive all their nutritional requirements from a single source – breast milk. It is indeed a unique source of nutrition, whose benefits are much emulated but never substituted by any other food source. Yes, it is true that if the mother consumes any undesirable food, it is reflected in her milk. But still it is considered much superior any formula you can buy off the shelf in a supermarket.

The World Health Organization (WHO) recommends that babies should be exclusively breastfed for the first 6 months. For the next 2 years and more, the baby should be fed breast milk and other appropriate nutritional food.

The American Academy of Pediatrics (AAP) also makes the same recommendation. The AAP recommends that in the first year of a baby, it should be compulsorily fed breast milk. In that one year, the first 6 months should be solely on the mother's milk.

These recommendations by the world's top health organizations cannot be brushed away. In this chapter we shall take a look at the various benefits of breastfeeding for babies that have been proved time and again by countless studies conducted by researchers and organizations worldwide.

Benefits during the first few years

The breast milk being the most ideal combination of nutrients, babies who are well fed on breast milk display much higher immunity to diseases and ailments than babies who are not. The following are some of the benefits that children derive in the first few years of their life when breast milk was the staple of their for an year or more;

- First and foremost, breastfeeding drastically brings down the incidence of Sudden Infant Death Syndrome (SIDS). This has been observed by researchers in Third World countries, where SIDS is a huge threat to the longevity of infants and is a major contributor to the child mortality rates in such countries.

- Numerous studies have indisputably proved that the immune system is strengthened and fortified as a result of breast-feeding. When the mother nurses the baby, antibodies from the mother pass on to the child, thereby boosting its immunity. Examples of this are the immunity against diseases such as tetanus, diphtheria, whooping cough and influenza against which the mother would have taken vaccination. Breastfed babies also show a much better antibody response to vaccines than babies who are raised on formula food.

- The chances of the baby contracting any respiratory disease are vastly brought down when the baby is raised on its mother's milk instead of any supermarket formula. In fact, studies have conclusively proved that the infants who are depraved of breast milk have a three times higher risk of severe respiratory ailment compared to infants who had consumed breast milk for at least for the first 4 months of their lives.

- Infants who are formula fed run a risk for diarrhea, three to four times higher than breastfed infants.

- Researchers have proved that the incidence of infections in the ears, nose and throat and the ENT canal are reduced by a great margin in babies raised on breast milk. This is a very important factor because, all over the world, ear infections are one of the primary reasons why babies fall sick and have to be administered antibiotics.

- Although the Western society and developed world does not face the issue of child mortality, it is still a much-prevalent menace in most parts of Asia, South America and Africa. And it is a widely known fact that babies who are formula fed stand a very small chance of living past their first year. Take for instance the South American country of Brazil, where the mortality rate of a baby raised in formula is about 14 times higher than that of a breast fed one.

- Another great benefit of breast milk is the immunity it grants against common allergies. Children all over the world suffer from susceptibility towards allergies, caused by causative agents such as pollen, dust, insects, citrus fruits etc. It has been noted by various researchers that a good one and a half years or more of breast-feeding can improve the resilience against such common allergies. Another fact that has been observed is that when the parents suffer from any allergy and when their baby is breastfed, the baby invariably becomes immune to those allergies.

- It has been undeniably proved that the ability of your baby to withstand infections and diseases in the first few years of its life is magnified if you breastfeed it for at least the first 6 months without break.

- Breastfeeding makes the baby more intelligent. It contains a multitude of poly-unsaturated fatty acids, which are an integral nutrient for the proper and wholesome development of brain. It has been proved in studies that the cognitive development of your baby is enhanced if it is fed breast milk for at the first one or two years. Short and sweet, breastfeeding makes your baby more bright and intelligent.

- Breastfeeding drastically brings down the risk of any wheezing problems manifesting in the child.

- It is said that one amongst every five children in the world an ailment called Eczema, a dermatological condition where the skin becomes itchy and dry in areas. This can be prevented to a large extent by breastfeeding.

- Infants who have been fed exclusively breast milk for at least the first six months show a much better resistance towards developing Type-1 Diabetes Mellitus.

- Researchers have also noticed a much lower incidence of the disease called Necrotizing Enterocolitis in breast fed babies. It is a medical condition in which the necrosis or tissue death is observed in portions of the digestive tract in premature infants. This is an extremely lethal condition, which is the second biggest reason for infant mortality throughout the world.

Benefits later on in life

Not all benefits of breastfeeding are visible when the child is still an infant. Yes, it is true that a lot of the advantages are visible in the infancy but there are a lot of other benefits that manifest later on during the life.

- Researchers have proved that children who were sufficiently breast fed in their infancy are much less likely to develop to Type -2 Diabetes Mellitus later on in their life. In fact, the chances are 34 percent less than formula fed infants.

- Dental health also improves in case of children who were breast-fed. There are many studies that correlate breast feeding and dental health.

- Obesity is another condition that is observed much more in children who were formula fed in their infancy. Breast fed infants stand a 20 to 30 % lesser risk of being obese later on in their life.

- Breastfeeding also protects your child against cancer to a great extent. Many recent Oncological studies have shown that infants who are raised on formula are 8 times more likely to develop some sort of cancerous growth in their body before they turn 15, than breastfed babies. However to gain this immunity, babies should be breastfed for a solid year or more, with breast milk being the exclusive food for the first 6 months and for the rest of the period, being the predominant source of nutrition.

- Recently many studies have shown that people who were breastfed as infants show a much lower incidence of hypertension or other blood pressure ailments. Here again, as in the previous point, this marked immunity was noticed in people who were raised on breast milk for the first 1 or 2 years of their infancy.

- As mentioned earlier, the cognitive development in a child is accelerated and gets on the right track when it is fed sufficient breast milk in its in infancy. This is reflected in the later periods of its life. Most psychological, learning and behavioral problems noticed in children can be avoided to a great extent if they are fed breast milk instead of formula. In fact so much is the effect of breast milk on mental health and acumen that some researchers have even found correlations between breastfeeding and personality traits such as maturity of thoughts, assertiveness, self-confidence etc.

- Many studies have proven that breastfeeding drastically reduces the incidence of Celiac disease especially when the nursing mother's diet was rich in gluten.

- Researchers have also found that the benefits of breastfeeding can be noticed in the form of reduced occurrence of cardio vascular diseases and cholesterol issues.

- A research paper selected by the United Nations Children's Fund (UNICEF) has, based on extensive controlled study, propounded that the perfect "U" shape of the dental arch prevents any sleep related problems such as snoring and apnea. And such a dental arch is commonly noticed in people who were breastfed well in their infancy.

Chapter 13

Breastfeeding for Twins, Premature and Adopted Babies

Breastfeeding her baby can be a very joyous activity for a mother and the joy will only double in volume if she has twins.

But feeding one baby can be hard enough and trying to feed two can be twice as tough. But by doing all the right things, you will be able to satisfy both your babies and they will have a chance to avail their fair share of milk.

Breast feeding tips for twins and multiples

- The very first thing that you must do to prepare for massive feeding sessions is to take up a feeding class. This will be important, as a qualified instructor will be able to teach you how you can efficiently feed your twins and the best positions that you can adopt. You might not get the time to join the class once your twins or multiples are born and so, you can join the class in advance if you have been told that you will have twins or multiples.

Getting your partner to join you in class will help him assist you while you feed.

- The internet can be your best friend when you want to clear any doubts that you have with feeding twins and multiples. You can find a lot of useful websites such as WebMD and La Leche League International, which will contain genuine information on medical topics. You can also do a specific search and seek answers to your problems or direct your question or queries to La Leche League International.

- You can also join a support group or a group of mothers who have twins and multiples, as you will have an insight into what it will take to feed two or more babies at one time. You can also make a friend there that you can call for help any time that you need it.

Types of positions for twins and multiples

- Double clutch. The double clutch position is one of the easiest and most widely used in the world as it is convenient for both the mother and the babies. In this position, the mother sits upright and places a pillow on both her thighs. She then places the babies on the pillows and their legs run around her. They are then made to latch and fed. This position is simple to get into and comfortable enough for long hours of feeding. But remember that the babies need to have their heads on the pillow and not be up as that might cause your nipples to ache and strain their necks.

- Double cradle. The double cradle position is the next most preferred for twins and multiples, as it is easy for the mother to cradle both babies. To attain this position, both babies are cradled inside folded hands and the baby on the right is made to latch the right nipple and the baby on the left is made to latch the left nipple. This is convenient for all three as the babies will have a comfortable resting position and the mother can adjust their height by moving her hands up and down.

- Cradle plus clutch. The cradle and clutch combination is just as convenient as the other two positions. This can be alternated with the rest two for a change in position. To attain this pose, place your babies on your lap and cross their legs over yours. This will ensure that they attain a proper latch and you prevent nipple pains.

Note: For multiples, you can assign a specific order.

Producing enough milk for twins and multiples

- Many women wonder if they will be able to produce enough milk to supply to their twins and multiples, but don't worry, as your body will be capable of producing enough milk, and more, for as many babies as needed.

- The key is to feed them right after birth and then as often as possible. This will cause your breasts to produce milk consistently and the more you feed, the more your body will produce.

- You can choose one baby for each breast and maintain the same order all throughout. You can help your babies feel comfortable by choosing one of the potions mentioned in the previous segment.

- Although there is no easy way to tell whether your babies are getting enough milk, you can always have your doctor check your babies' weight to assess whether they are of the right weight. If they appear lighter than necessary, then you need to feed them more often. You can also check their nappies to assess if they are getting enough milk and check their bowels for the same.

Breast feeding tips for premature babies

- Often times, feeding a tiny premature baby can seem like a herculean task. The baby will have to be cared for intensively, as he or she will be quite weak and in need of nourishment.

- When your baby arrives early, your body will produce special milk that is loaded with more vitamins and nutrients than for a regular baby. So you must, at any cost, feed your premature- this life giving milk- and help your tiny baby recover faster.

- Although there are formulas available just for premature babies, it is important that you use them as supplements to your own milk, as they will have a weaker immune system and remain highly susceptible to infection.

- If your baby is quite premature, then you will not be able to feed him or her directly and might have to pump the nutritious milk. For this, your nurse or doctor will provide you with the pump and the milk will be administered to the baby through a nasogastric tube.

- In a few weeks' time, your premature baby will be ready to nurse at your breast. But they will not be able to suckle enough milk and so, you will not have a complete drain. To tackle this problem, you must pump milk after your baby has finished nursing to help your body create more milk.

- Another hurdle that you will need to overcome is to teach your premature baby to suck swallow. They will not be able to do this as their minds will be too young and immature. You must allow them to suck and then tilt them a little to help them swallow. This will cause them to develop the habit and in 8 weeks' time, when the baby will gain normalcy, then he or she will not need any swallowing help.

- Remember that your premature baby is still very week and to help him or her conserve vital energy, you must feed them as soon as they are hungry. If you are negligent and your baby starts crying out of hunger, then they will end up wasting a lot of energy, which they will need to direct towards their growing. It is ideal to feed a premature baby every 3 hours as that is when they mostly feel hungry.

Breast feeding tips for pregnant mothers

- If you are pregnant with another baby and have a toddler to nurse, then don't worry, as all three of you will not have any risks.

- Your body will continue to produce milk just as well and there will be no difference in the quality or quantity.

- If you are having sore and aching nipples because of a fluctuation in your hormonal levels then you can decide to wean. Continuing on might leave your nipples sore and painful and cause problems for your next baby.

- Most mothers stop feeding their toddler when they are 6 months pregnant as managing a toddler on the pregnant belly can be quite tough, and might cause your unborn child discomfort.

- If in case you do deliver a baby and still have a young toddler to feed, then you must prioritize and feed your new born first as they will need to intake the colostrum. You can then feed your first child.

- To produce enough for both babies, you will have to consume healthy foods and double up on the liquid intake. Rehydrate yourself every hour and consume lots of fresh fruit juices.

Producing milk for adopted babies

- Adopted babies will also need to be fed breast milk as they are, after all, infants. But for a woman who has not given birth to a baby or never been pregnant, it might be difficult to induce lactation.

- However, with the right techniques, it is possible for all women to produce milk and for this to happen; you can talk with an expert. You must consult a breast milk expert as well as a pediatrician, as they will know how women can start to produce milk.

- The amount of milk that a woman can produce for her adopted baby can vary as per her body and also depend on how much the baby is nursing. It choosing to breast feed an adopted baby is one of the best decisions that you will make for both you and your baby as you will be able to establish a deep connection with him or her and they will develop a strong immunity.

- But it will be important for you to have a reasonable expectation out of how much milk can be produced. You might be able to supply enough or your baby might have to be supplemented with formula. It will completely depend on your body time. Some women decide to start inducing lactation before they adopt a baby as it will help them start feeding right away.

- The time taken to develop breast milk can vary between 1 month and 1 year and even if you have started your baby on solid food, you can still decide to nurse them.

- One of the best ways to induce lactation is to get your partner to suckle you, as your body will respond best to it.

You can also choose to stimulate your breast by pressing it for a few minutes every hour.

- If you wish to use a pump to induce lactation then make sure that it is efficient and of good quality as that will help you induce lactation faster.

- Some women decide to take up hormone therapy to induce lactation as it can be a sure shot way to produce milk. But these induced hormones can tamper with your body's hormones and so, you might have to consider the pros and cons of the treatment.

- One great alternative to hormone therapy is to consume natural plant based supplements that help in inducing lactation. Some herbs such as fenugreek, fennel and nettle root can help in inducing breast milk. You can consume these fresh or consume capsules or tablets that contain them to help you start lactating. But remember that these will only work if you are supplementing them with physical stimulation.

- You must continue consuming the supplements as they will help you produce more milk and maintain a consistent supply at all times.

- The Supplemental Nursing System is a boon to mothers with adopted babies as they will have their babies at their breasts and will be able to supply enough and more milk. The system calls for pumped or formula milk placed inside a pouch and hung around the mother's neck. A thin tube that runs from the pack with one end of it placed on the mother's nipple. The baby will be able to latch to the mother's breast and draw from both her nipple and the tube.

Human milk banks

- Human milk banks are meant for babies that are adopted and their adoptive mother is not able to produce any milk. They are approached if the baby is not responding well to formula either.

- Some babies will start to throw up when fed formula and can also develop allergies. In such situations, they simply have to be fed human milk and one good source for it is human milk banks.

- These are places where mothers donate milk for other infants and it will be safe to administer it to your baby.

- If there is no human milk bank in a pediatric center near you, then you can search for one online.

- But remember that buying milk from milk banks can be quite an expensive affair, as they will only have a limited quantity. So you can check with your insurance company if it will cover your expenses.

If you feel that it is very expensive for you to afford, then as a last resort, you can look for a nursing mother, who will help nurse your baby. This will ensure that your baby gets his or her, due, first milk and the danger of infection and other problems can be avoided

Chapter 14

Breastfeeding for Working Mothers

Working mothers might have to return to work after a few months of giving birth, but that should not stop them from feeding their infant. It is important for the infant to be feed for at least 6 months and more is always good.

In this chapter, I will talk about the various things that you can do for your baby, to prevent any disruptions in his or her feeding schedule.

Pumping

Pumping enough milk to last your baby 5 or 6 hours is the best thing for working mothers. Pumping milk and storing it will allow your baby's caretaker to feed your baby and you can work freely. You can buy a good quality electric breast pump, as that will make it easy for you to pump, as also help you be assured of the quality that will be fed to your infant. Another advantage is that electric pumps pump faster and so, you will have the chance to pump more milk if you start pumping early in the morning. Just make sure you store it in the correct way and instruct the caretaker the right way to feed.

Expressing milk

Expressing milk refers to removing the breast milk that would have accumulated over the course of the day. Remember that you will have to return home and feed your baby fresh milk, and for that to happen, you must remove as much as you can. You must remove the milk at all the exact times as you would feed your baby and make sure that you try and completely drain it each time. For an 8 hour job, you can pump out every 2 or 2 and a half hours as that is how often you usually feed your baby. It might take you about 15 minutes to pump each time and so, you must try and not have any work assigned to you when you decide to pump.

You can carry your electric breast pump to express your milk out. It can be quite tricky to find privacy but you can talk to your boss and have a private room arranged for you. There are specific guidelines that tell companies to not assign new mothers the bathroom to express their milk as it can be quite unhygienic. You can use a conference room or an empty office cabin or even the store room if there is some space in there. Avoid rooms such as the generator room or some other room where there is heavy machinery as you might feel uncomfortable. As long as there is privacy and an electric outlet to plug in your pump, you should be good to go.

Whatever milk that you pump can be stored for later use.

Taking breaks

If your house is close to your office, say a 5 or 10 minute drive, then you can ask permission to go feed your child at least twice a day. You can ask your boss if it will be feasible for you to leave for no more than 30 minutes each time and get back to work. This will help you work well, as you will get a chance to be with your baby and not worry about him or her. Besides, it is not a trend that will continue forever and might only last a couple of months. If you think your baby's nanny will be able to bring your baby to the office every alternate day or so, then that will also work. You can feed your baby in the same private room where you pump milk.

Visiting play school

If your child is in playschool, then you can transport your expressed milk to the playschool and have his or her caregiver feed them. You must make sure the playschool is close by and that it will not take you any more than 10 minutes. If you have more time on your hands then you can feed your toddler and return back to office.

Tips to pump milk in office

Sometimes the work environment might not be a conducive place for you to pump your breast milk. You might feel conscious and this can cause you to struggle with it a little. To help you pump better, here are a few tips that you can undertake.

- Remain as relaxed as you possibly can and don't fear being seen. If you are extremely conscious, then you can lock the door to the room and pump in peace. But there is really no need to feel shy as pumping breast milk is a natural process.

- To help pump out more milk, you can lightly press your breasts and massage the tips. This can also help pump it out faster.

- You can listen to some calming music and close your eyes to visualize your baby, and that he or she is suckling you.

- If you need help with the visualization, then you can look at a picture of your baby or carry along their belonging like a small toy, a pacifier or a bib. It will help you pump faster and better but don't get carried away and start crying.

- If you can carry your laptop to the expressing room, then you can continue working while your milk is being pumped. That way, you will be able to leave home early and not be behind in your work.

Chapter 15

Basic Tips and Facts on breastfeeding

In this last chapter of the book, we will look at some of the basic tips about breast feeding that will help you feed your baby in a proper way.

- For mothers who are chain smokers, it is important to quit smoking as soon as possible. If you are slowly decreasing smoking the number of cigarettes in a day, then you can continue to feed your baby, as your milk will help your infant combat any respiratory problems. Remember to never smoke in your baby's vicinity and tell you partner the same. If you consume alcohol, make sure that you limit it to a bare minimum as over drinking can cause your baby harm. You must avoid doing recreational drugs at all costs as these can harm your baby to a very large extent. If you are having problems quitting, then you can check into rehab and not feed your baby until you are completely clean.

- Breastfeeding can delay ovulation to a certain extent but is not a sure shot way to prevent pregnancy. If you wish to have sex when you are breastfeeding your child, and do not wish to get pregnant, then it is important to use condoms. If you want to consume birth control pills, then you must check with your doctor first, as it can tamper with your hormones and might have a bearing on your milk production.

- You must avoid using heavy chemical laden cleansing products in your house. Although the risk of these being absorbed by your body and passing to your infant is not high, you still might have to consider it a threat. You can shift to natural essential oil cleansers for your house, bathroom and use eco friendly dish washing liquid or bar to cleanse your dishes. Even with your baby's bottles, nipples and other such equipment, you must not just sterilize it but also wash it with a chemical free cleanser. The same extends to chemical laden cosmetics and creams.

- Some mothers might suffer from post partum depression, which can cause them to feel irritated and not be in a good mood. This might cause their body to not produce enough milk, as they will suffer from excess stress. For this, she might have to consult with the doctor and maybe see a psychologist. Although long lasting depression is rare, it might be important to treat even the occasional blues, as the mother's emotional make up will have a large bearing on the quality and quantity of milk that she produces.

- Making use of a pacifier is a great idea to teach your baby to latch on to your nipple the right way. You can make use of one, when the baby is a month old, but make sure you use good quality and age appropriate pacifier. Once the baby starts suckling the pacifier, he or she will relate it to your nipple and suckle you with ease. They will know when to stop and drink until they are full.

- Your infant will need quite a bit of vitamin D to help develop strong bones. For this, you might have to give them a vitamin D supplement or take them out in the sun for a short while, as your milk alone might not fulfill the requirement. You can also ask your baby's doctor for help and suggest a good supplement.

Chapter 16

Breastfeeding ABCs

In this chapter we shall give you some tips that will ensure that your breastfeeding experience is as enjoyable and pleasant for you and the baby as it is scientifically and technically correct. There are plenty of tips floating around on the internet and of course let us not forget the pretentious aunt who professes to know everything that is to know about breastfeeding. However let us not get flummoxed by any of that. The tips mentioned below are based out studies and researches conducted by experts in a thoroughly scientific fashion. So without further ado let us proceed.

The ABCs

Every nursing mother should know the ABCs of the breastfeeding.

Awareness - Be aware of your baby and his actions. This is imperative because when it comes to feeding your baby, it is just you and your baby. Know the signs and actions by which the baby tries to convey that it is hungry. For example actions such as hands moving towards the mouth, suckling sounds and cupping movements with the lips. Please do not wait for the baby to cry and wail.

Be patient - Patience is a virtue in every walk of life and it applies to motherhood too; especially when you are nursing. Be patient when your baby is suckling, let him/her take all the time they want.

Comfort - This is the most important factor. If you are tensed and hurried it will affect the flow of milk too. Therefore before you begin breastfeeding, make sure that you are comfortable and relaxed. Support yourself with sufficient pillows and cushions when you sit or lie down to nurse. Play some music that is soothing and slow. All these will contribute towards ensuring proper flow of milk.

Positions

The position of nursing plays a significant role in ensuring that the breastfeeding is comfortable for both the mother and the baby. Whatever be case, neither you nor the baby should be strained. Mentioned below are three of the most comfortable positions.

The cradle

One of the most favored positions amongst mothers worldwide is the cradle position. Hold the baby in such a manner that the baby's whole body faces you and his head is resting on the inside of your elbow. Make sure the baby feels supported by positioning its tummy against your body. Now, you can either wrap the head and neck of the baby with your other hand or support its back longitudinally by taking your arm between its legs.

The Football

In this position, you support the full weight of the baby in a single arm. And because of this, this position is most suitable for newborn infants and small babies less than a few months old. Hold the baby in such a fashion that your forearm supports the baby diagonally, with your palm being the support for its head and neck, like how you would hold an American football.

Cross cradle

The cross cradle is a position that is quite popular owing to its use in feeding babies with a weak suck. Some babies will not be able to latch to their mother's nipples well enough and so, taking up this position will help better that state. To get into this position, you can rest your baby on the opposite arm of the breast that you are using and support your baby's neck with your palm. This position can be quite comfortable for both mother and child.

The side lying

As implied by the name, this involves you lying on the bed on the side with the baby next to you. Use the free hand to help the baby latch on and then use that arm to secure the baby so that it may not twist or turn much. This position is great for nursing at night before sleeping or when the baby wakes up hungry in the midnight.

Chapter 17

Weaning

Weaning is the process by which the baby is gradually taken off its diet of breast milk and is introduced to other foods that are generally consumed by adults. Correct and timely weaning is as significant as ensuring a correct process of breastfeeding because of its physical and psychological implications and repercussions. In this chapter we shall discuss 2 key concepts regarding weaning. We shall look at what is the right age for weaning and then subsequently we will provide you with some techniques for weaning your baby off breast milk.

The right age

The right age for weaning depends on a lot of factors such the culture, the atmosphere at home, the physical condition of the baby and the mother etc. The developed countries generally frown upon breast-feeding for anything more than 10 to 12 months. Whereas in developing countries in the Asian and South American region, many mothers consider it natural to continue breast feed till the baby is 2 to 3 years old.

If you recollect what was mentioned earlier in this book, the American Association of Pediatrics and World Health

Organization advocate a diet to be followed for a minimum of 6 months, which is exclusively breast milk. However if you don't feel uncomfortable with it, you could continue breastfeeding for a little over one and half years, since breast milk being a part of the diet is highly advised. At the same time you could begin introducing baby foods from the 7th or 8th month onwards.

Techniques for gentle weaning

Given below are some techniques that you can follow for gently weaning your baby. Understand that this is a gradual process that can take a few months to be effective, and not an overnight phenomenon. Hence make sure you have the right mindset for this.

- The preliminary step is to ensure that the baby will get sufficient nutrition from other sources. This is why it is important to introduce new things into the menu once the child is 7 to 8 months old.

- Do not offer and do not refuse. This applies to those babies who just do it because you offer them. When the usual time for nursing comes, just move on with your chores. If they ask, then indulge them, but repeat the same step the next day.

- Do not wear clothing that is tight fitting or which has a low neck. This is because the sight of your breasts may wake the longing in the child to be breastfed. You have to be careful about this factor for approximately a year after your child id weaned.

- The common tendency of mothers to nurse their babies after they have hit themselves somewhere or have fallen down to placate them should be avoided. Teach your child to hug you and cry to deal with the pain rather than suckling.

- Be aware that some children may not make a smooth transition into adult food and may resort top tantrums, and crying bouts to have their way. Deal with this and be compassionate yet firm.

- Give alternative choices. For instance, when it is the usual time for the toddler to be nursed, show some alternative tasty food and encourage it to try them out.

- Reduce the duration. This is one of the most effective techniques. By this time your child will already be eating alternative food and is just suckling due to habit. Gently reduce the duration of nursing the next time. And the times after that reduce further. This way you can slowly wean him/her completely.

Conclusion

I want to thank you again for choosing this book!

I sincerely hope this book was able to help you learn more about breastfeeding, how important it is for you and your baby, the bonding it leads to, why you should pursue it and build your confidence when it comes to producing more milk for your child.

The challenges of breastfeeding can be endless and almost every new mother faces a different predicament every time. If you cannot seem to find support on your breastfeeding journey in your immediate environment, then look for other means such as seeking advice from a lactation consultant, a breastfeeding advocate pediatrician, or an online group dedicated solely for breastfeeding mothers. You might be surprised to learn that you are not alone in your journey. Don't let a few struggles compromise the best nutrition you can give your child. All these problems have a solution and all you need to do is seek help in the right places.

The next step is to take your personal journey as a learning experience and pass it on to other breastfeeding mothers. Encourage others to opt for this book and help them learn more about breastfeeding. Let more mothers know that it is not supposed to be easy and that it gets better in time. Remember that children will only nurse on you for a year or two (more for others) and after that, they will wean and outgrow it. You will surely miss holding them close to your heart, so enjoy every minute of it.

Thank you and good luck!

Check Out Other Books
by Misty Jordyn

Mindfulness: Healthy Living with Low Stress, No Anxiety or Worry, Created through Spiritual Mindfulness and Meditation, Peace and Happiness

Insomnia Natural Remedies: The Guide to Eliminating Sleeplessness and Insomnia with Natural Treatment

Infertility: Get Pregnant Fast Cookbook: Women's Health, Fertility, Homeopathy, Cookbook, Pregnancy, Baby Health, Healthy Living

Infertility: Get Pregnant Fast Exercise Guide: Infertility, Fertility, Get Pregnant, Pregnancy Exercise, Fertility Exercise, Healthy Living

Infertility: Get Pregnant Fast: Women's Health, Fertility, Homeopathy, Cookbook, Pregnancy, Baby Health, Healthy Living

The Bladder Pain Cure- The Quick Guide to Naturally Treating and Preventing Bladder Pain, Interstitial Cystitis, and Bladder Infections

The Chronic Pain Cure- The Step by Step Guide to Natural Chronic Pain Relief and Treatment

Childbirth: Natural Childbirth Labor and Delivery: Natural Childbirth, Holistic, Home Remedies, Pregnancy, Infertility, Healthy Living

Back Pain- Effective Natural Back Pain Relief and Remedies

Breastfeeding: A New Mom's Comprehensive Guide to Breastfeeding: Pregnancy, Motherhood, Childbirth, Pregnant, Healthy Kids, Healthy Children, Nutrition

Essential Oils as Natural Medicine- The Guide to Essential Oils and Natural at Home Remedies for Better Health and No Side Effects

Thyroid Disease- Naturally Heal Your Thyroid and Manage Hyperthyroidism and Hypothyroidism

information is without contract or any type of guarantee assurance.

The trademarks that are used are without any consent, and the publication of the trademark is without permission or backing by the trademark owner. All trademarks and brands within this book are for clarifying purposes only and are the owned by the owners themselves, not affiliated with this document

Disclaimer Notice

Please note the information contained within this document is for educational and entertainment purposes only. Every attempt has been made to provide accurate, up to date and reliable complete information. No warranties of any kind are expressed or implied. Reader acknowledges that the author is not engaging in the rendering of legal, financial or professional advice.

By reading this document, the reader agrees that under no circumstances are we responsible for any losses, direct or indirect, which are incurred as a result of the use of information contained within this document, including, but not limited to, -- errors, omissions, or inaccuracies.